Pu
Stickm
129 Broadway,
StickmanC

Copyright © 2019 Stickman Co
The right of Hannah Ens   author
of this work has been asserted by her in accordance with the
Copyright, Designs and Patents Act 1988

All rights reserved. This book is sold subject to the condition that no
part of this book is to be reproduced, in any shape or form. Or by way
of trade, stored in a retrieval system or transmitted in any form or by
any means, electronic, mechanical, photocopying, recording, be lent,
re-sold, hired out or otherwise circulated in any form of binding or cover
other than that in which it is published and without a similar condition,
including this condition being imposed on the subsequent purchaser,
without prior permission of the copyright holder.

Cover design and Illustrations by Hannah Ensor

Printed in Great Britain by
Grosvenor Group (Print Services) Ltd, Essex.

A CIP catalogue record for this
book is available from the British Library
ISBN 978-0-9927217-2-5

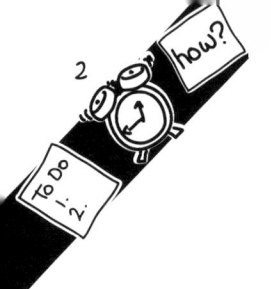

Disclaimers:

Every condition, and every person is different. What works for one person may not work for another.

This isn't a book of rules, it's a book of things to consider in case they help.

Discuss changes in condition management with an appropriate health care professional before trying them.

Advice from stickmen won't cure medical conditions, but it might make those conditions easier to live with.

Foreword

When I started working with people who live in chronically uncooperative bodies, I set myself the career goal of putting myself out of business. I can retire when everything I teach is common knowledge, when all the misinformation about symptom management has been squashed, and proper, practical pacing is something you're taught when symptoms first start.

This book brings me one step closer to that goal.

Hannah has a wonderful way of imparting knowledge, her outlook on health and life is one that can only be learnt by years of experiences, both positive and negative. I sincerely hope that reading this will help people avoid some of the 'negatives' that Hannah (and I) learnt from!

**Jo Southall,
Occupational Therapist.
jboccupationaltherapy.co.uk**

Intro preface-y thing

By Hannah Ensor

Pacing is a key part of living well with my persistent pain and fatigue. It's not a cure, but it helps me get the most out of life in the body I have. But it wasn't always like this.

Pacing was initially explained to me as limiting myself on 'good' days to slightly more than I can manage on 'bad' days. The problem was that if I followed that rule, I'd never leave my bed!

Gradually my understanding of pacing evolved and changed due to advice and experience.

It changed my life.

This book contains the pacing tips and practicalities I wish I'd been told from the start.

Pacing is...

...a way of spacing tasks so you get the most from the energy you have. It is commonly used for conditions which cause persistent pain or fatigue. Instead of trying to push through symptoms and causing them to get worse, recognising what makes things worse and what helps, then using that knowledge to create a lifestyle that works for you.
Sometimes pacing can lead to long term improvements, other times it simply helps you cope with your symptoms. But either way, life with good pacing is MUCH more fun than

Boom and Bust!

Boom and Bust is....

...when instinct says "Quick, do everything and make the most of your energy" so we push until we splat under a mountain of symptoms. Each splat means recovery time. We loose strength, and stamina while we recover. On our next 'okay day' we 'Boom' again, but are less healthy than before, so we manage less and splat sooner. When this spiral is followed for long periods, we get worse.

Some of us try to keep pushing through the 'Bust'. The 'Boom' may appear to last longer, but the 'Bust' is even more severe. This is equally unhelpful, and can cause a similar overall worsening.

The good news is that we don't have to stay in this spiral! Pacing can get us out - so carry on reading for some top pacing tips.

The boom and bust spiral:

- Yay! Feeling okay-ish!
- Must do everything!
- Must push through...
- Splat
- Total flop.
- Feeling a bit better.

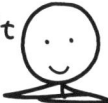

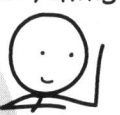

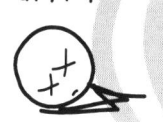

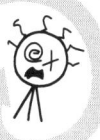

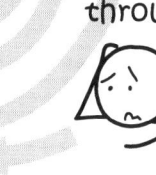

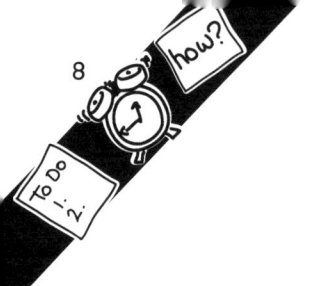

First:
Get to know your body.

We can't manage symptoms which we don't recognise or admit that we have. Variable symptoms and/or years of being told we're imagining symptoms make this harder, so this will probably be an ongoing process!

9

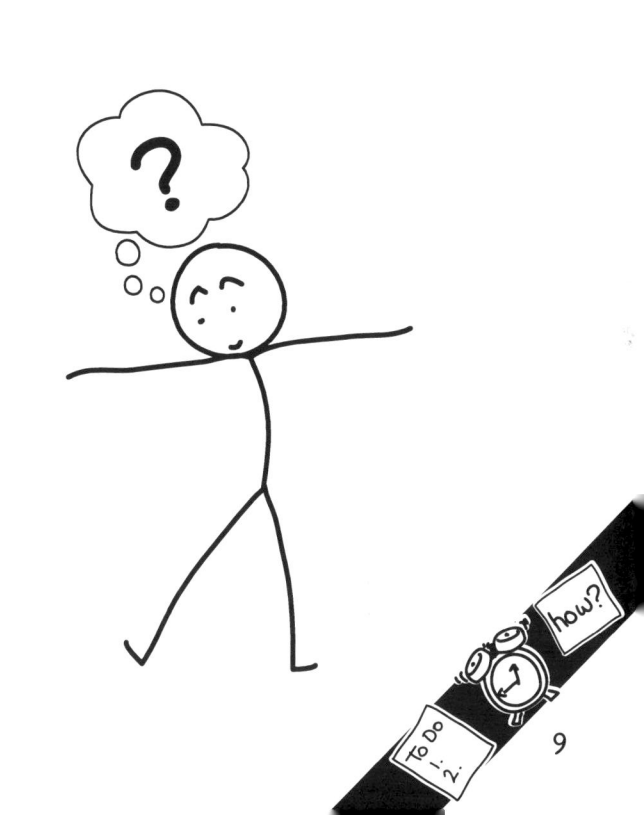

10

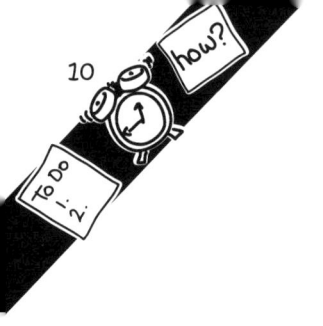

List your main symptoms.

Not all your symptoms. That would be long and boring. Focus on symptoms which get in the way the most. This list may change over time.

11

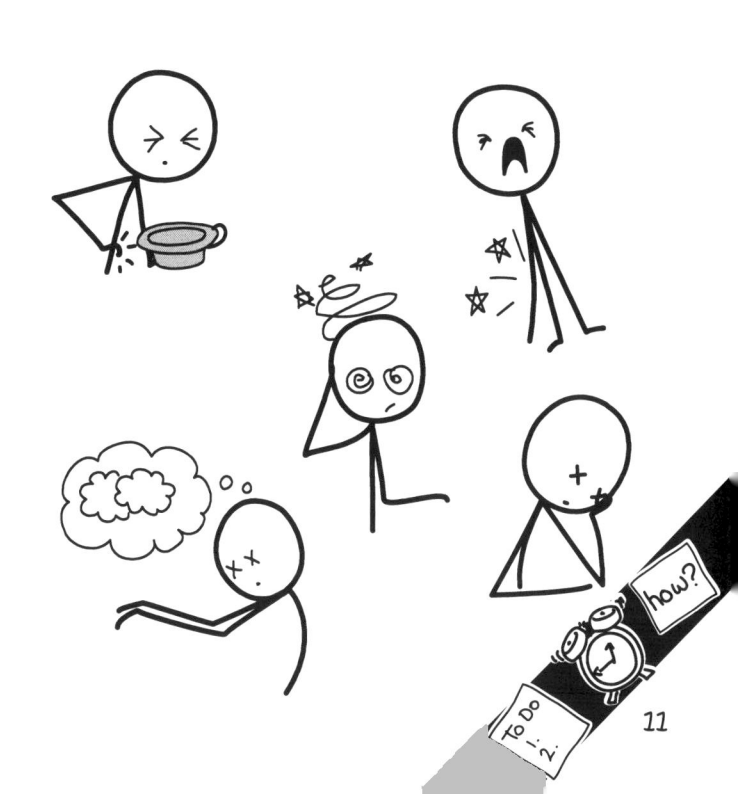

12

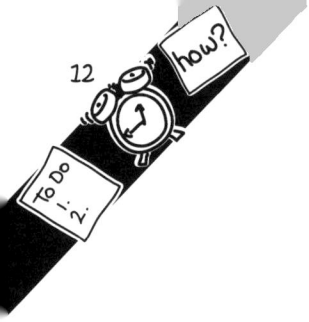

List the things that make those symptoms worse.

This will include things you can control (sitting, talking, concentrating, dehydration, rushing etc.) and things you can't (illness, hormone levels, emergencies etc).

how?

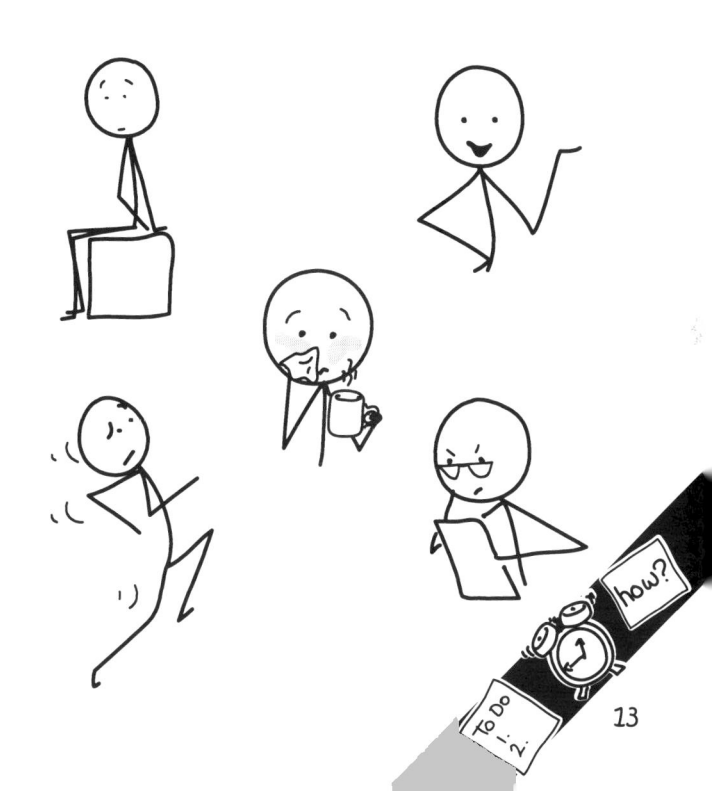

13

14

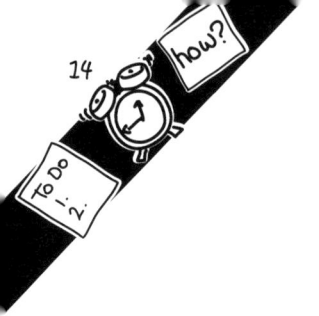

List the things that help those symptoms.

Heat/cold, medications, stretching, movement, relaxation, standing, lying down, exercise, distraction - anything that helps you.

15

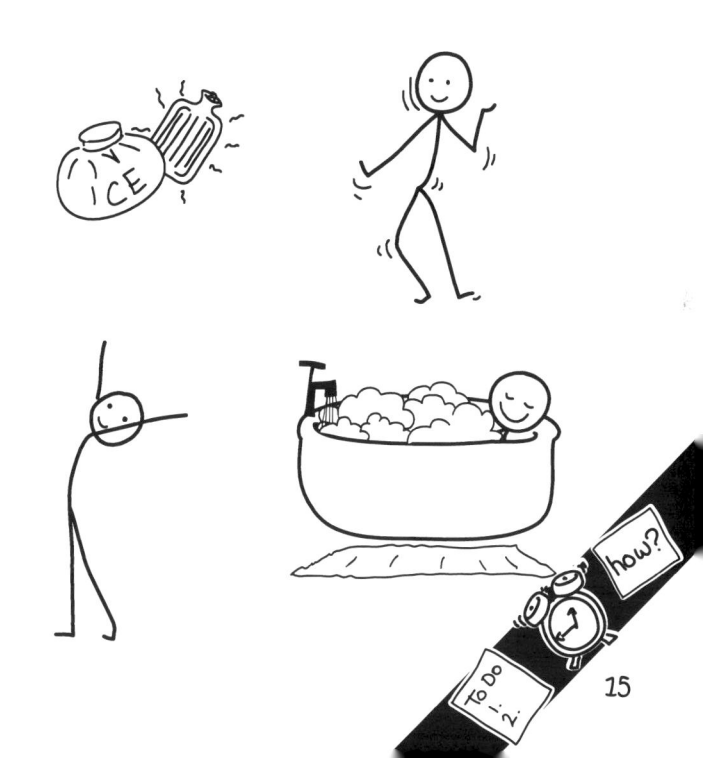

Keeping a diary, list, or mind map of activities and symptoms for a short time can uncover things that help and things that worsen.

Repeat this periodically because things change over time.

Keeping a diary showed me that sitting upright and still = utter exhaustion, but repeated wriggly sitting with a 30 minute limit = mild fatigue. It was life-changing.

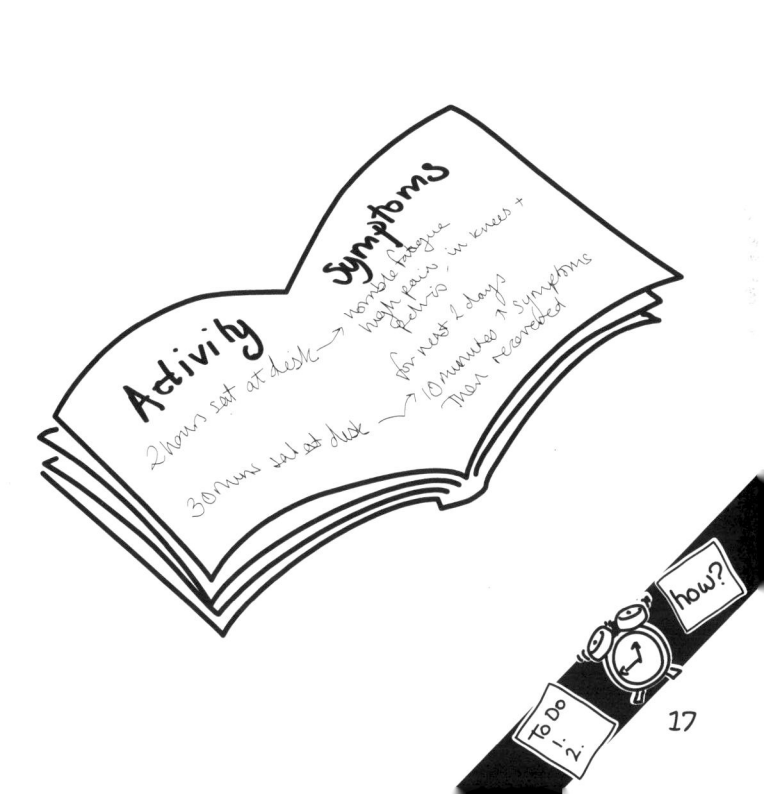

Activity	Symptoms
2 hours sat at desk	horrible fatigue, high pain in knees + pelvis, for next 2 days
30 mins sat at desk	10 minutes - symptoms then recovered

17

18

Once you've got to know your body a bit, you can start to pace using

the 3 Ts.

Task

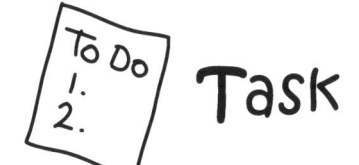

Technique how?

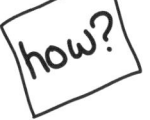

Timing

Task.

Think of all the things that need to be done in the next day, or week, or period you are planning. Writing them as a To Do list can help.

21

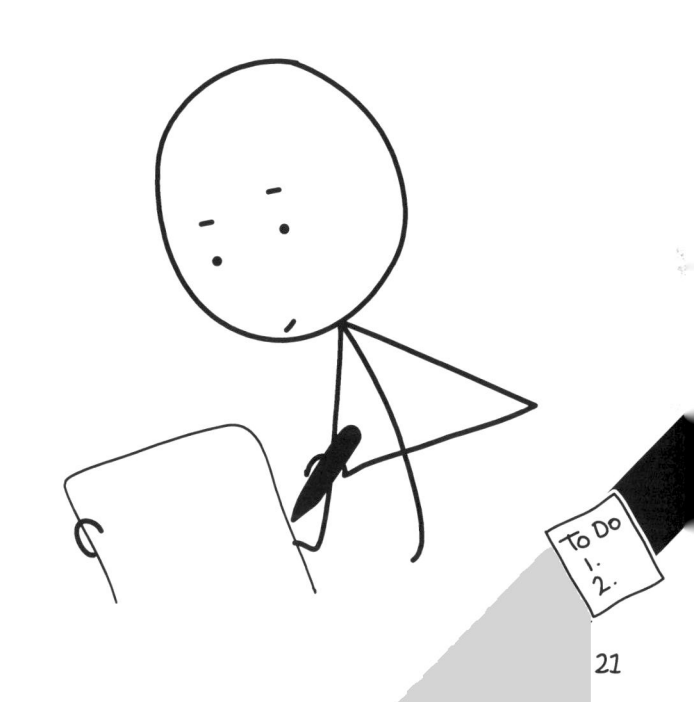

22 Task

Include everything.
Not just the impressive things.
Not just the ones you think 'other people' would think worthy of going on a To Do list.

If tasks like washing, dressing, preparing meals, and eating use noticeable energy, worsen symptoms, or are difficult: include them. No task is too small.

23

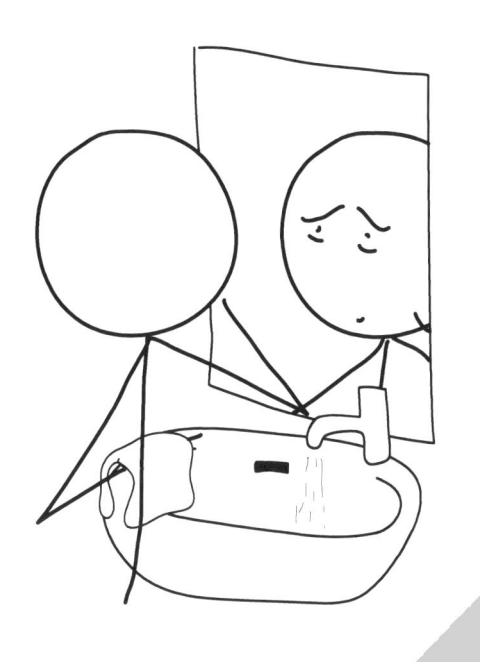

Task 24

Note how challenging each task is, based on how you are now.
Not how you were yesterday.
Not how you think you ought to feel!

It may help to colour-code tasks as red/amber/green for challenging/okish/easy, to make it easier to see where you might be expecting too much, and where you might be able to do more,

25

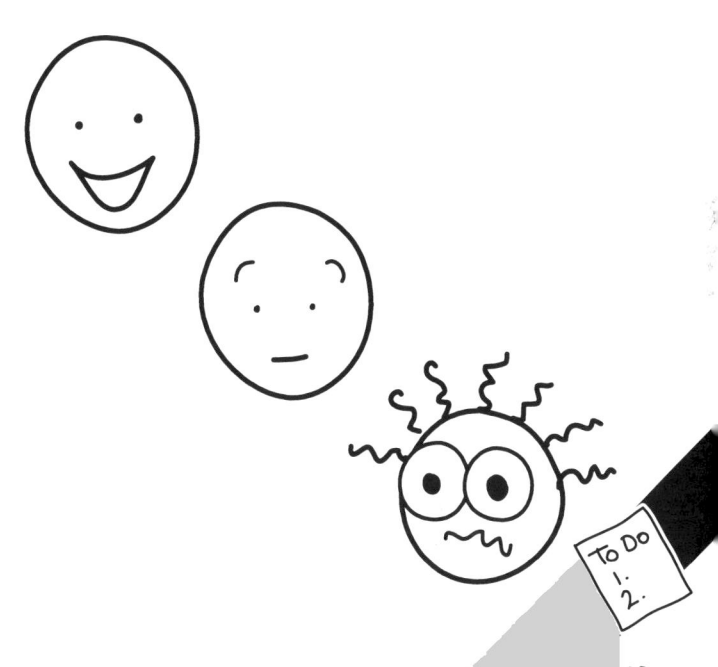

26 Task

Remember: Tasks requiring concentration can be just as challenging and exhausting as tasks requiring physical activity!

News flash: Not being able to see symptoms doesn't stop them being real.

27

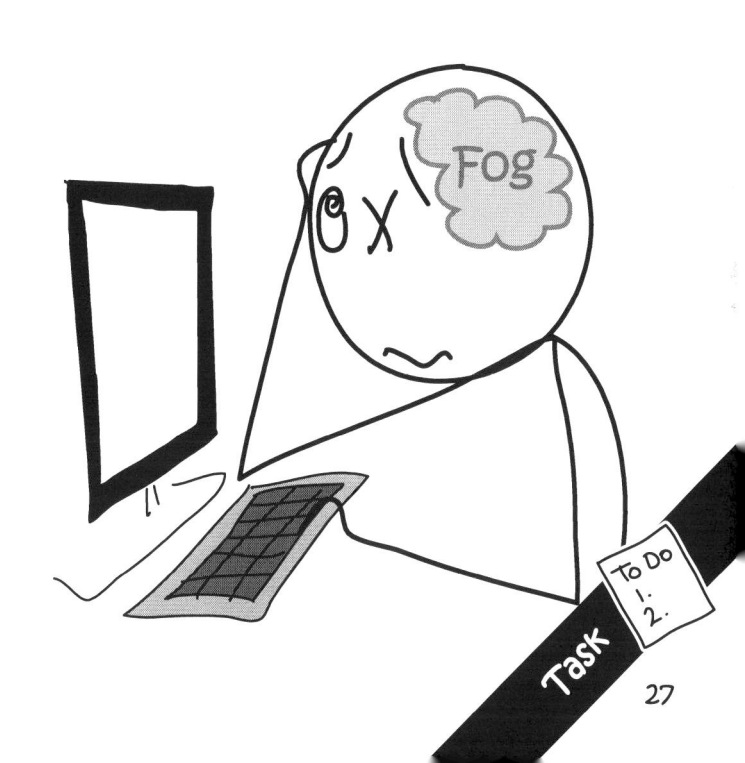

Task 28

Think up 'easy' things to do. Tasks that enable recharging.

Focusing only on challenging tasks feeds the Boom and Bust cycle, and the delusion that only 'challenging' stuff counts. Easy and recharging tasks are essential to getting the most out of life - so give them the high priority they deserve, and be proud when you do them.

29

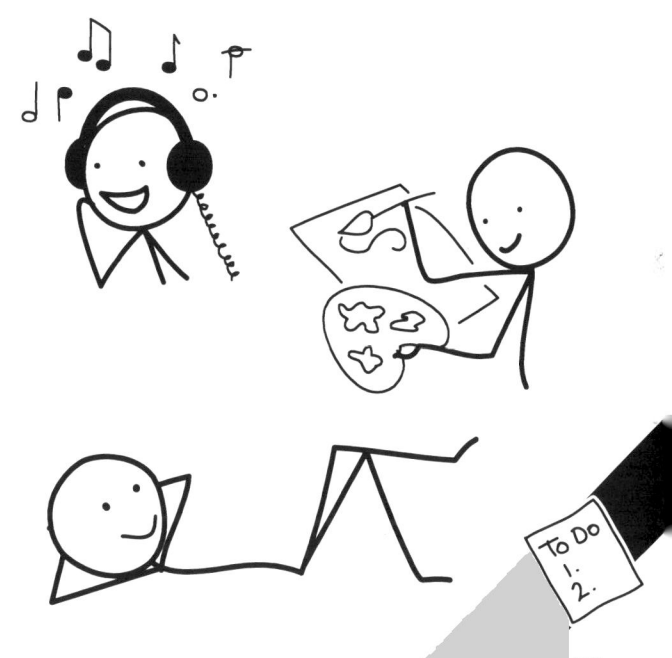

Technique.

How can you make tasks less challenging?

Think creatively and leave 'average' behind.

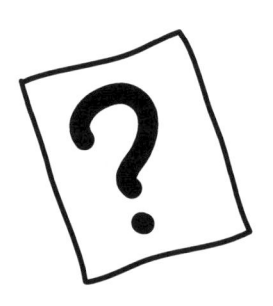

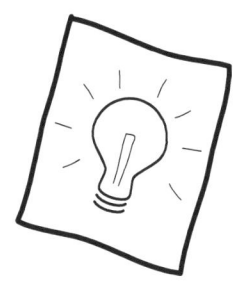

Think about Technique when:

- You need (or want) to do it, but it aggravates symptoms.

- You can do this task okay, but need to conserve energy for later.*

*Or any other good reason applicable to you.

Technique how?

Technique how?

32

Can you use something from your 'Things that Help' list to make a task less challenging?

Challenging includes painful, fatiguing, symptom-aggravating and so on.

Technique how?

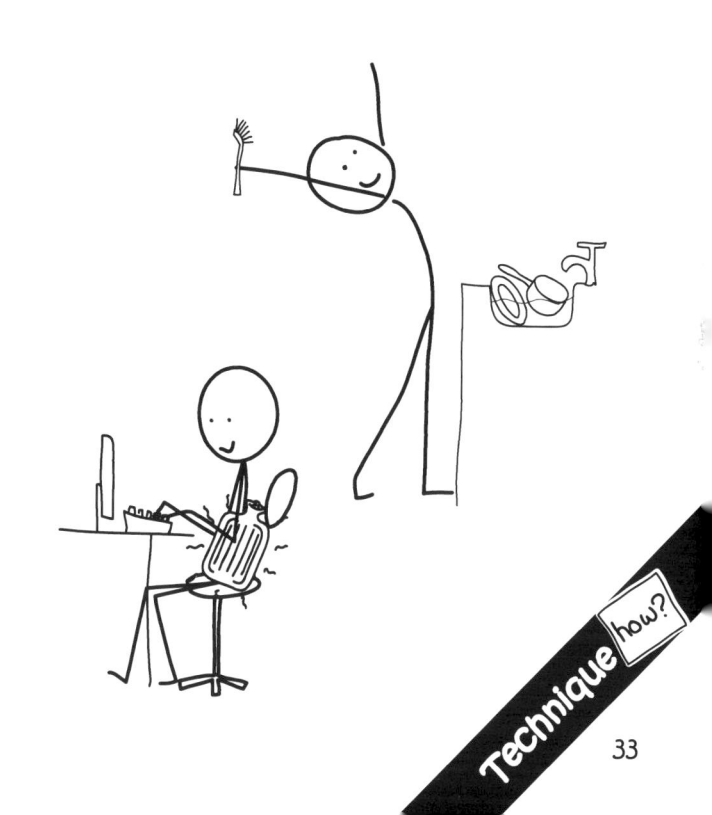

33

Technique how?

Could you use a different position?

- Sit instead of stand.
- Lie instead of sit.
- Switch position part way through.

Patient support groups with a pacing/self management focus are great places to find techniques that might work for you.

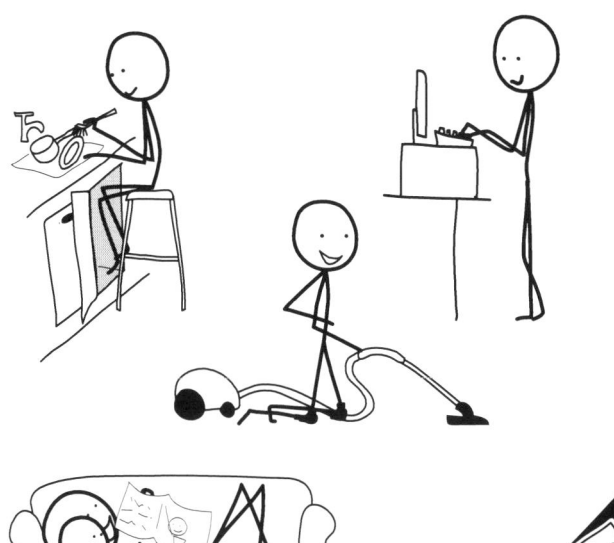

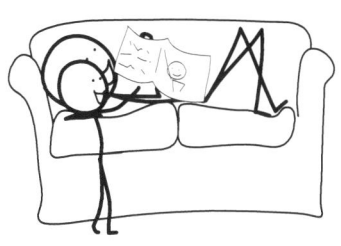

Technique how?

35

Technique how?

Or use a clever piece of kit?

> Ergonomic pens.
> Mobility aids.
> Voice recognition software.
> Grabber.
> Trolley.
> Knee pads.
> Gym ball as a seat...

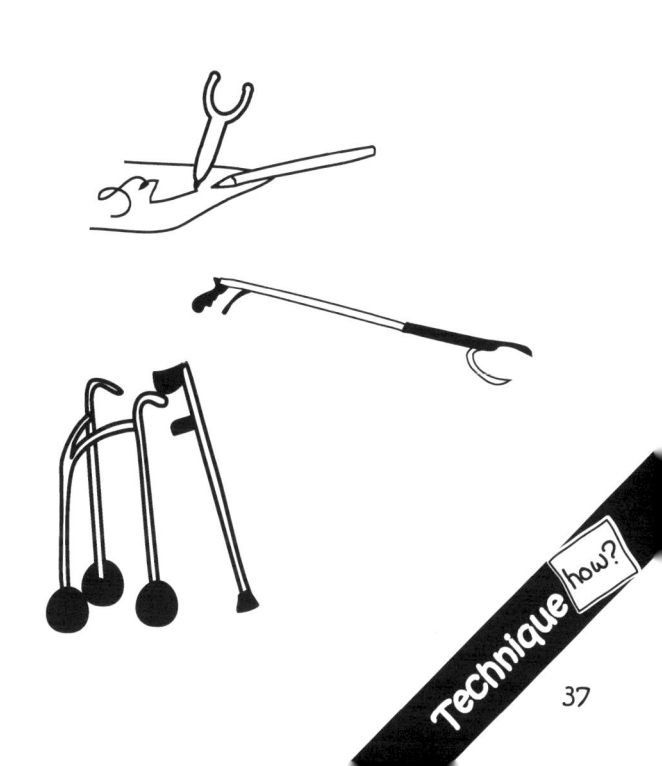

Technique how?

37

Technique how?

Or some other cunning plan?

> Pre-prepared veg.
> Bulk cooking on quieter days to create home made ready-meals.
> Employ a cleaner.
> Only wear non-iron clothes.

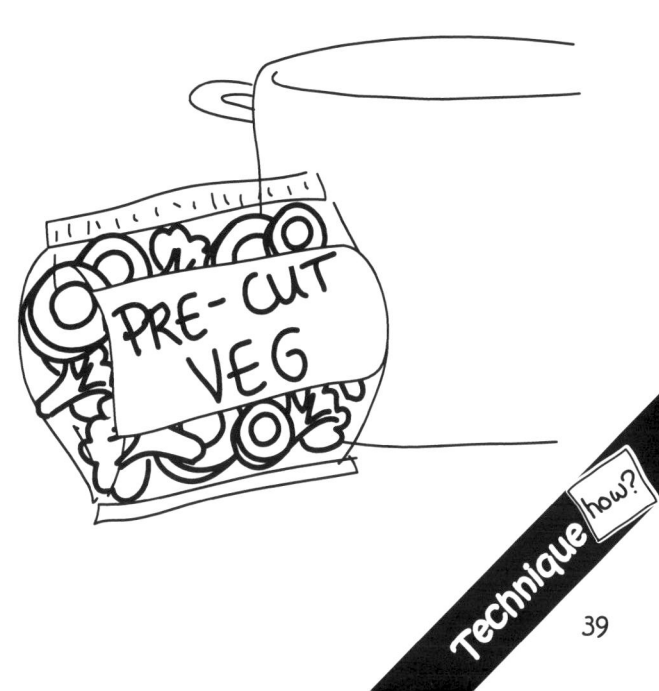

Technique how?

39

Technique how?

40

Note:
Braces and mobility aids can help manage pain and fatigue, but over-use will mean muscles get weaker. Weaker muscles mean more pain and fatigue in the long run, so use them wisely!

A leaflet about appropriate splinting is available from StickmanCommunications.co.uk. It is hypermobility focused, but is applicable to many protect & weaken / use & aggravate dilemmas.

To splint or not to splint?

That is the question.

Whether 'tis nobler in the joints to suffer -

The slips and twinges of outrageous laxity,

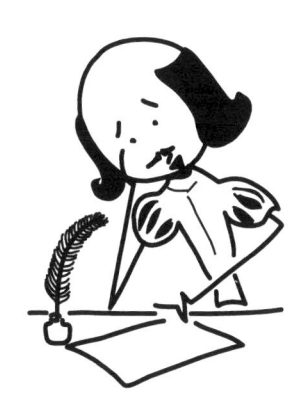

Or to brace limbs against a sea of troubles

And by supporting them, to rest -

    to weaken.

(Inspired by: William Shakespeare)

Timing.

What needs to be done today?

Does it have to be done at a specific time?

How long will it take?

Might a time limit on an activity help?

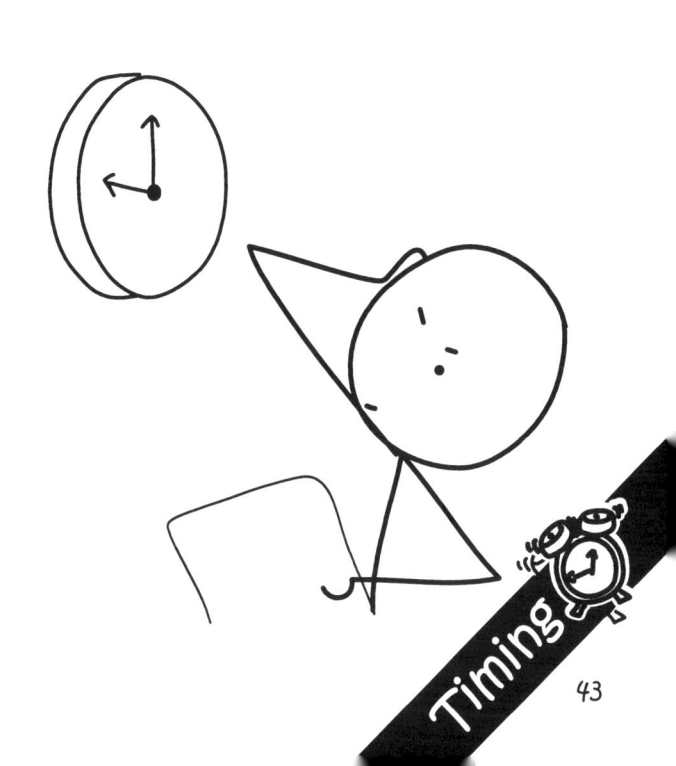

Timing

43

44 Timing

How long a task takes will affect how challenging it is.

Do you need to do it all at once?
Splitting a task into small sections can help.

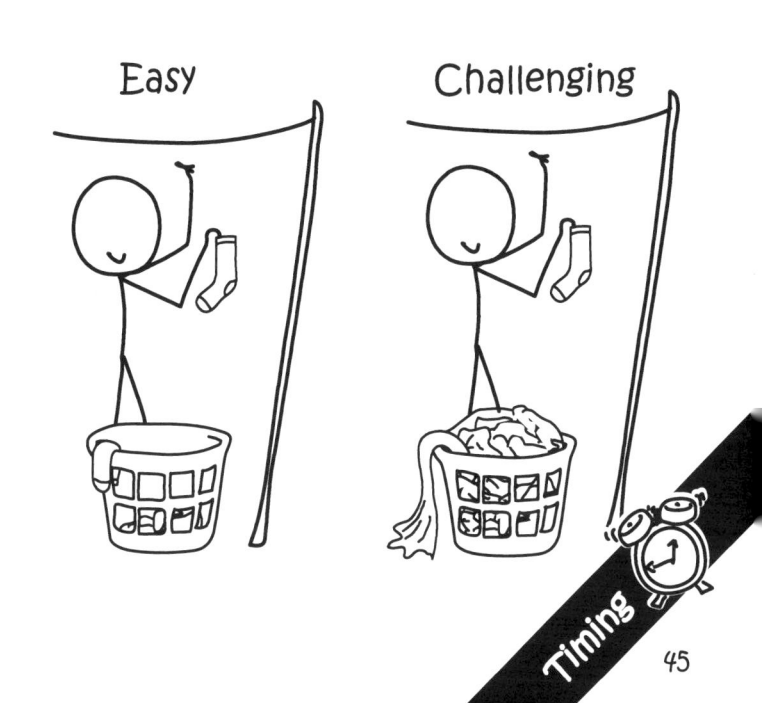

Timing

45

Timing — 46

Swapping Task or Technique before your body forces you to stop can reduce recovery time. Over a longer period, it may even increase how long you can do a task without triggering symptoms!

e.g. If you can sit for 8 minutes before brain fog kicks in, aim to swap after half that time - 4 minutes. You can gradually increase this time as you feel able, but remember: the aim is to manage symptoms, not test endurance!

Recovery takes minutes.

Recovery takes months.

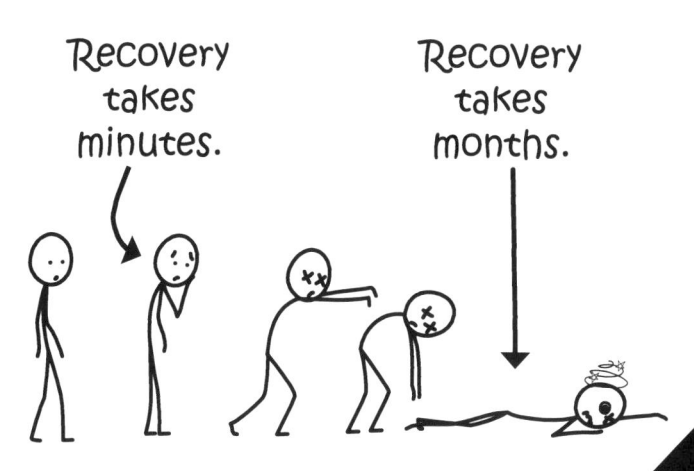

It feels much nicer to decide to swap rather than total flop being constantly forced on you by your symptoms.

Timing

47

48 Timing

Use a timer to remind yourself to swap task or technique.

Remember: Success is **not** about doing tasks despite the symptoms. Success is swapping task or technique when the timer goes and having fewer or more manageable symptoms.

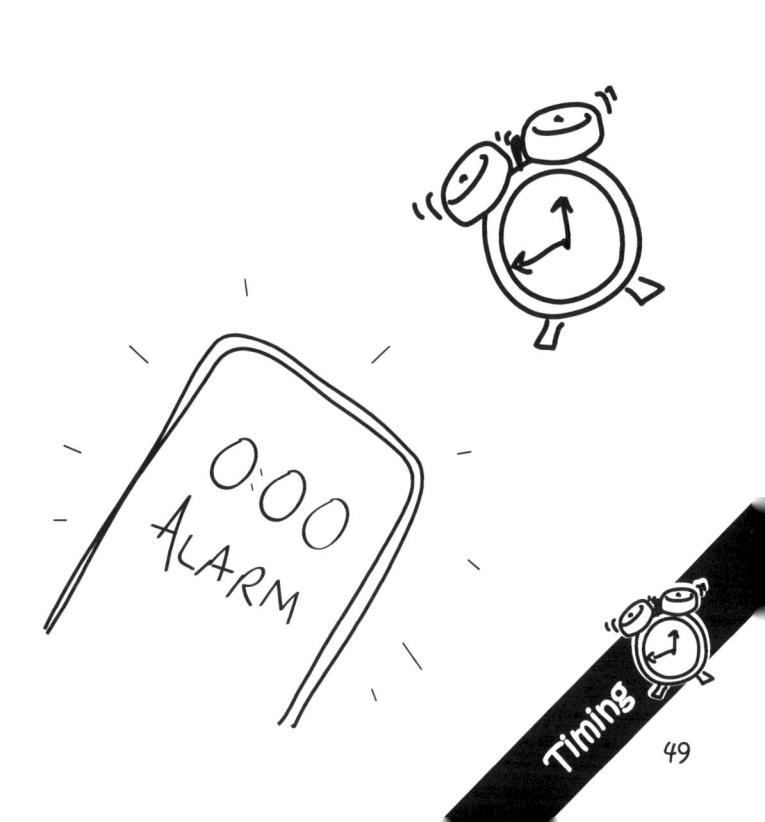

Timing

49

50 Timing

Where possible, swap to something which challenges a different part of you while allowing the tired part to recharge. Then go back to the original task later.

Examples:
Walk part of the distance, sit and make a phone call, finish walking the distance.
Hang washing out for 3 minutes, sit and reply to an email, hang more washing out for 3 minutes.
Clean the kitchen floor, sit and fold some washing, sweep the hallway.
Sit and write, stand and do filing, sit and write.

Brain challenge

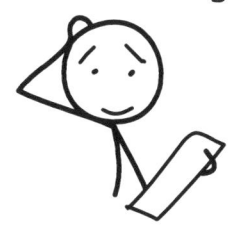

Leg challenge

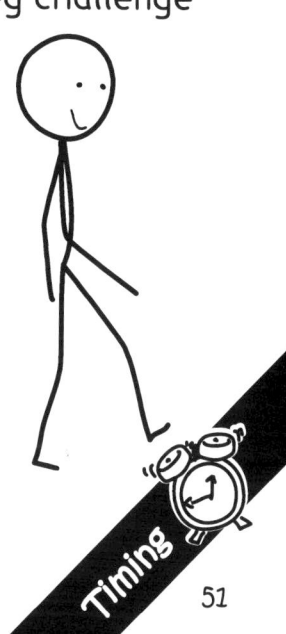

Hand challenge

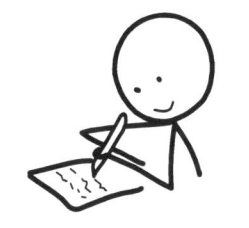

Timing

51

52 Timing

If you can't change the Timing, for example at work, school, or appointments, focus on Technique and what you schedule directly before and after the time-specific task.

Pre-charging

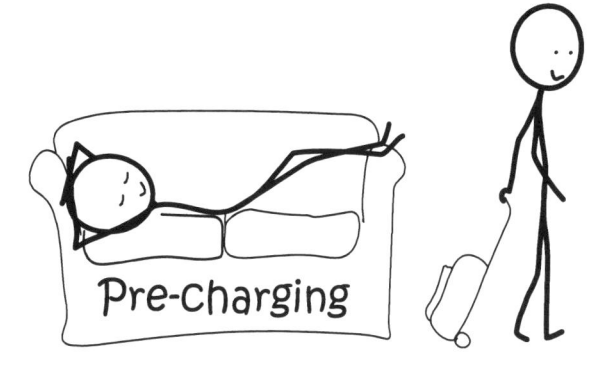

Timing

53

Technique how?

54

Are symptoms affected by meal times or other activities?

Do you need to allow recovery time as part of your schedule?

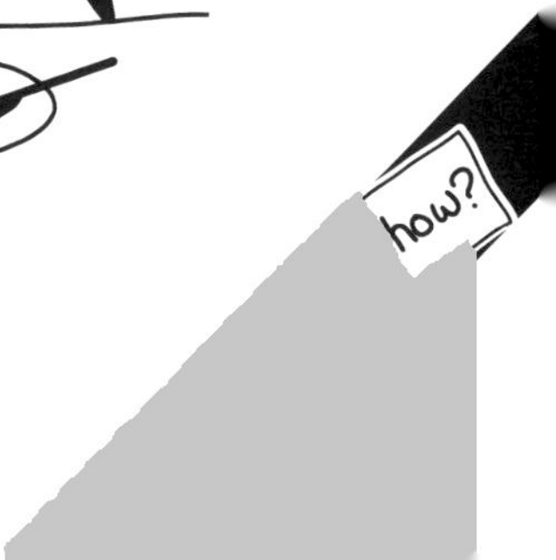

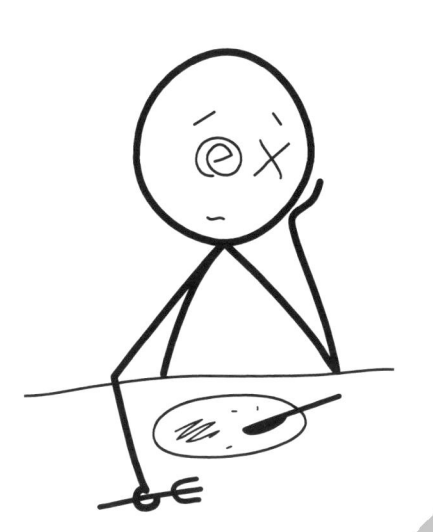

Timing

56

If something is important but always leaves you too tired to function, would it work if you did it just before going to bed?

Some people report that fatigued muscles mean more injuries and pain from everyday tasks, but doing exercises just before bed means getting the recovery time they need overnight - so they get stronger with no extra injuries.

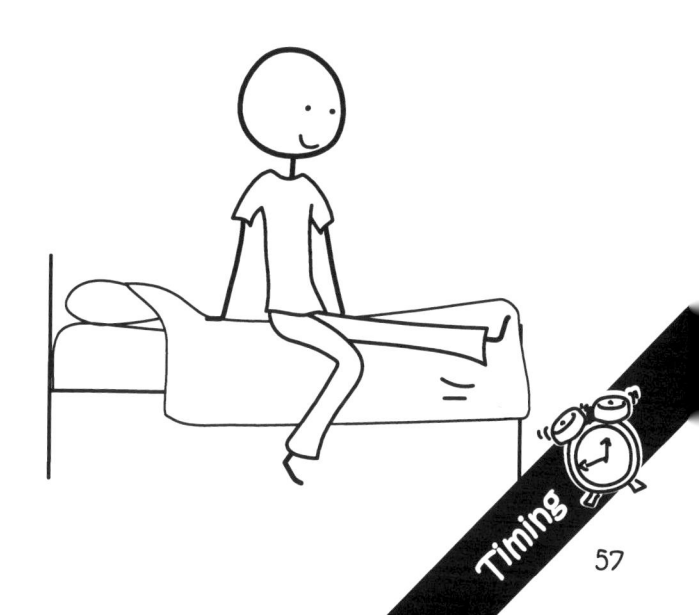

Timing

57

58 — Timing

Treat "I'll just finish this" with extreme caution.

It feels silly to stop - you are "in the zone" "nearly done". But in reality a short break when you need it can make all the difference.

Then you can do a few shorter, more effective, sessions instead of one long session struggling through the fog, pain, or other symptoms.

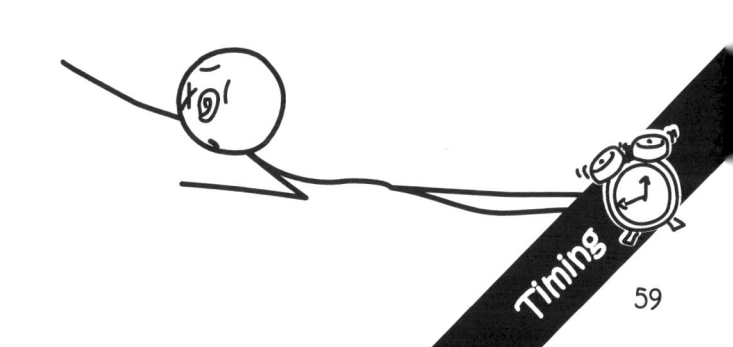

Timing

General Tips:

On a bad day the main activity might be resting, but there should still be swapping between different positions, and preferably a little movement rather than at total stop of everything. Even if it's just stretching or gently moving fingers and toes, or tensing and gently tensing and relaxing muscles.

61

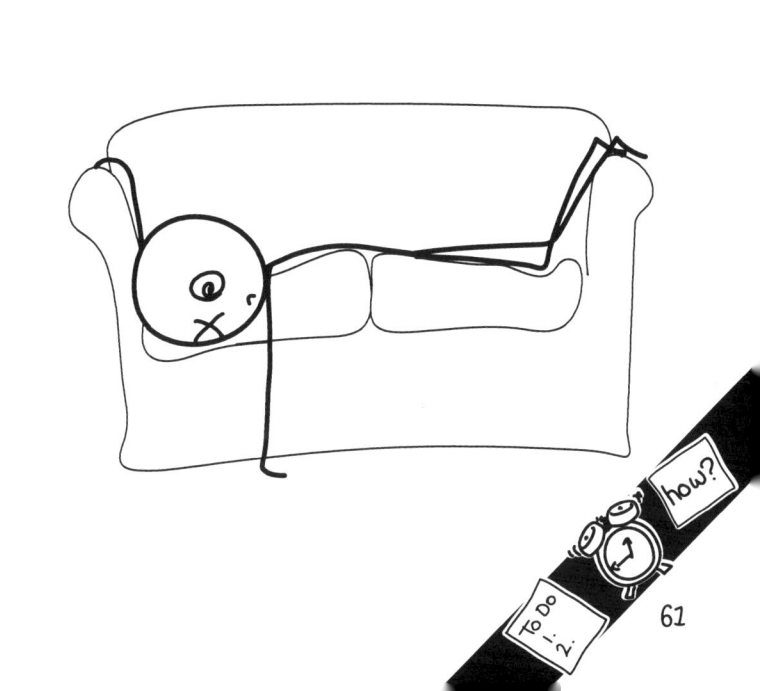

Make your pacing plan for bad days* in advance - a befuddled brain is not good at working out sensible pacing.

Following prearranged plans is much easier.

*Also called a 'Flare up' plan.

63

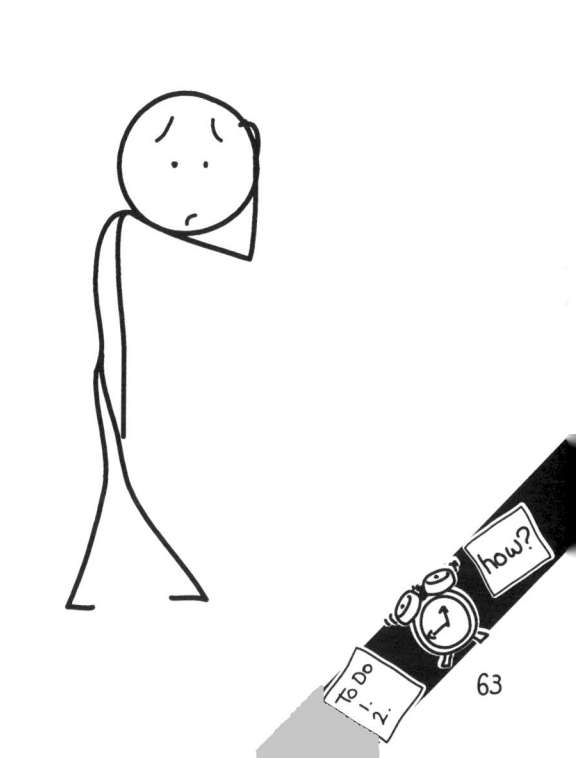

Have an actual box or cupboard with your 'bad day' stuff in it.

Include things that will help you through; a list of exercises/stretches, hot water bottle, blanket, medications, snacks, photos of loved ones, distraction - DVDs, crafts, puzzles, colouring etc.

If things (or ideas) can't be placed in the box, write them on a list and put the list in the box.

65

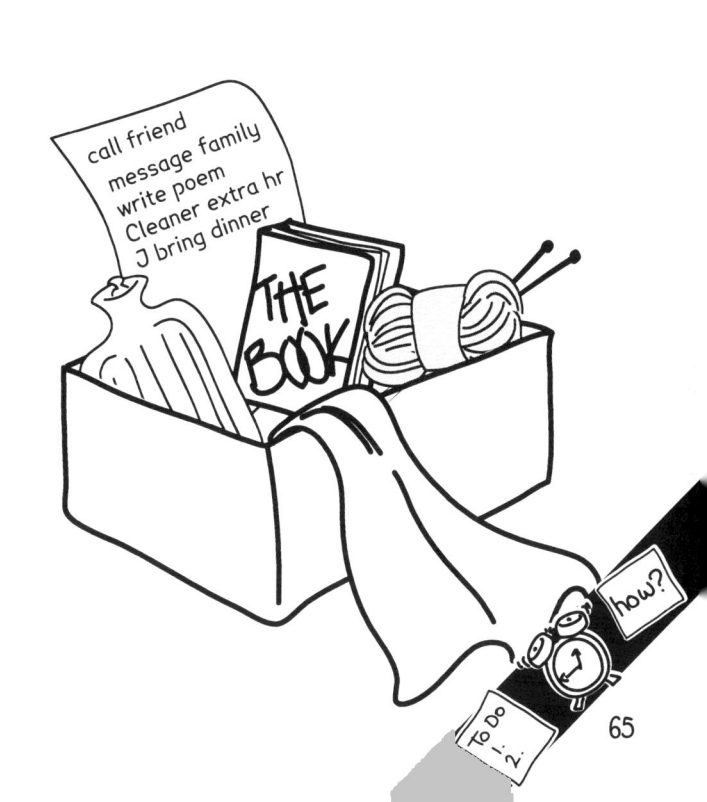

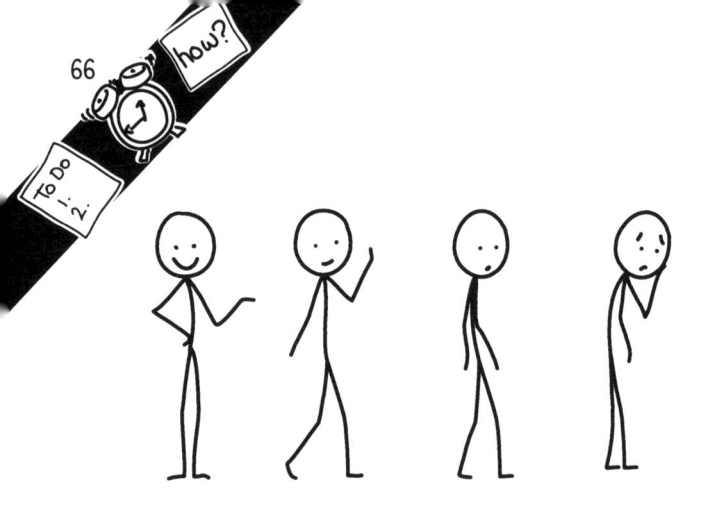

Learn to recognise (and respond to) the little symptoms as they start to build up.

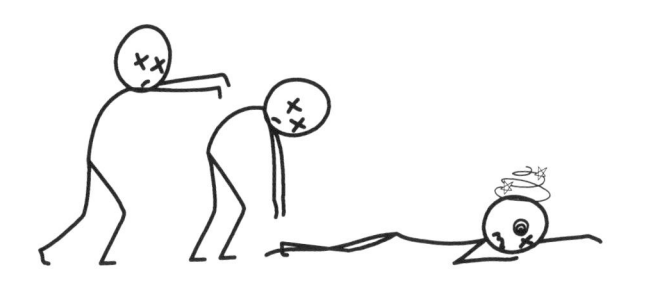

This will help you avoid prolonged splat.

Myth: "I ought to do that"

'Ought to' clouds our judgement. It is often based on unrealistic expectations - both our own and other people's.

It is a heavy, guilt filled burden.

Instead stop, think, and decide whether you are going to do it or not, based on how important it is to you, the likely consequences, and any other relevant factors. Perhaps you decide to do it, perhaps you decide not to, but either way it becomes your choice.

You are in control.

Which feels SO much better.

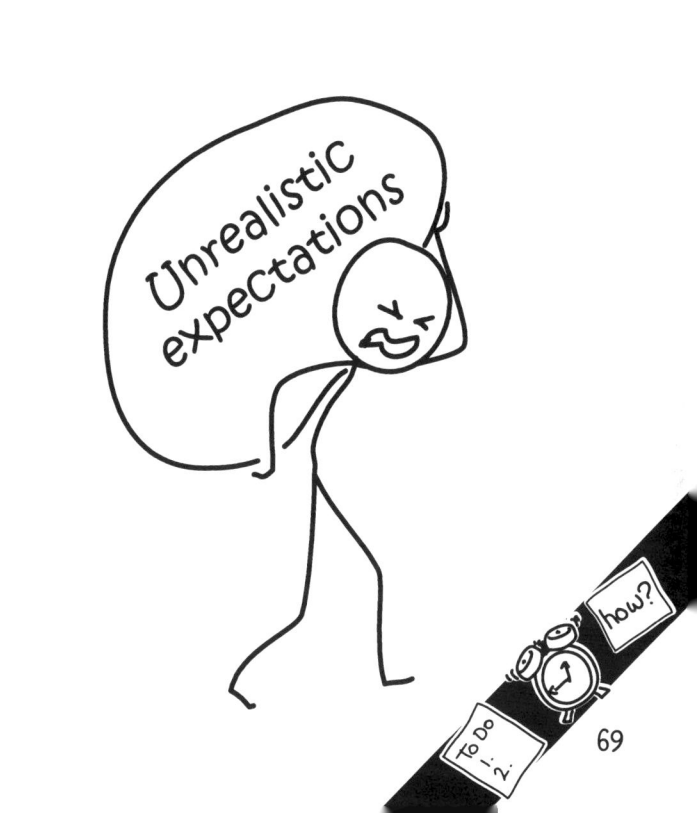

Timing

Myth:
"Find a basic level of activity I can cope with, and stick to it."

Find a level for bad days - use it on bad days. Be aware of that limit. But also learn symptom progression and on better days it is fine to do more - push gently while keeping an eye on symptom progression and make sure you don't slip in to 'Boom and Bust'.

For symptoms that don't appear until a day or two later, try to learn what factors affects them. A diary of what you did and your symptoms over the following few days can help you spot patterns which will help you pace.

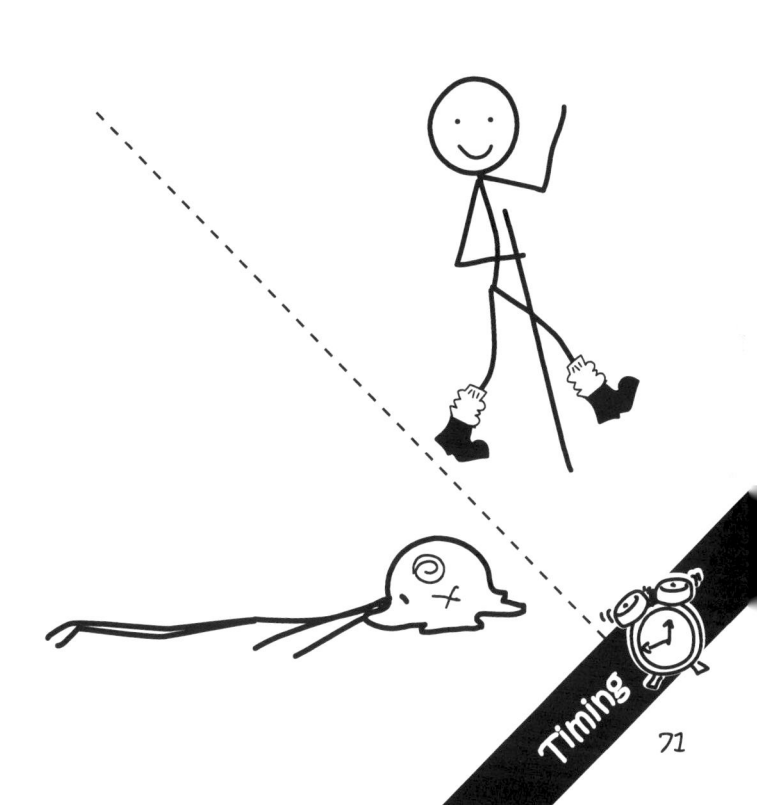

Timing

Myth:
"If I don't give 100% I haven't tried hard enough and am giving in."

Elite athletes only give 100% for special events (e.g. actual races) - after which they do less for a few weeks while they recover. In training, if they aim for 100% all the time they quickly get over-training injuries and performance worsens. This will happen to us too if we try to live at 100% all the time.

Stepping back when we still have a little energy left isn't failing - it is a wise and constructive approach to everyday life. Save the 100% for special occasions.

Everyday effort level

Special event effort level

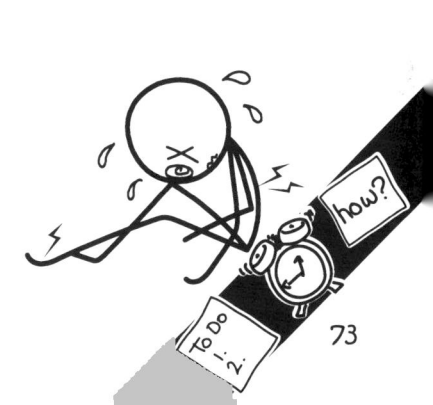

Beware of long term overdoing!

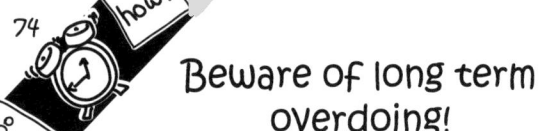

If symptoms are increasing over time, it's time to revisit pacing basics. Doing a little bit too much each day can feed a downward spiral without an obvious crash.

Where an underlying condition has got worse, better pacing will make life easier.

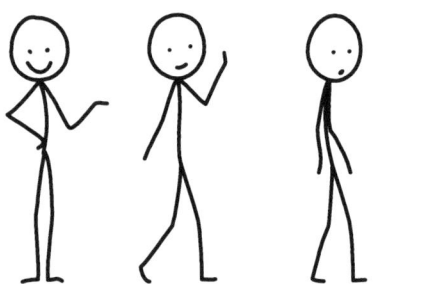

Where an underlying condition hasn't got worse, having some recharge time and then pacing back into the 'I can cope with this' range allows your body to recover, and may mean you can slowly build back up without triggering the same level symptoms.

Staying in 'overdoing' will almost always result in ever-worsening symptoms.

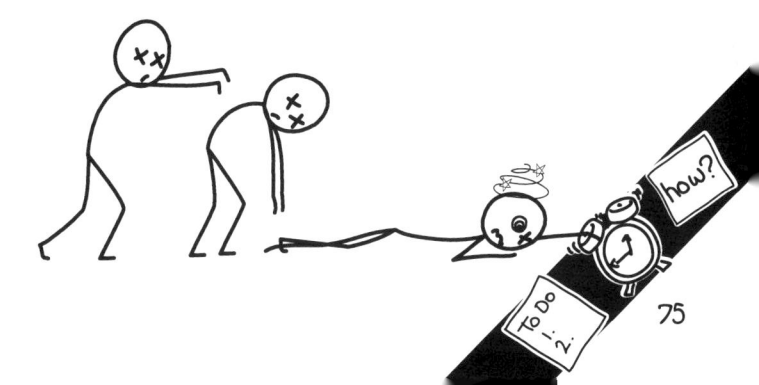

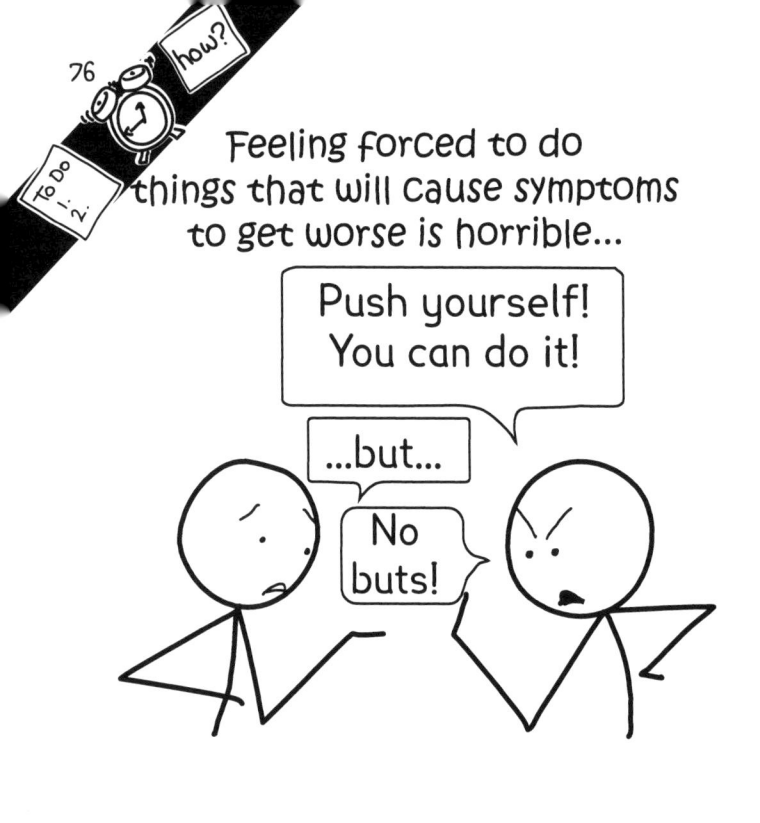

Feeling forced to do things that will cause symptoms to get worse is horrible...

> Push yourself! You can do it!

> ...but...

> No buts!

...however well meant.

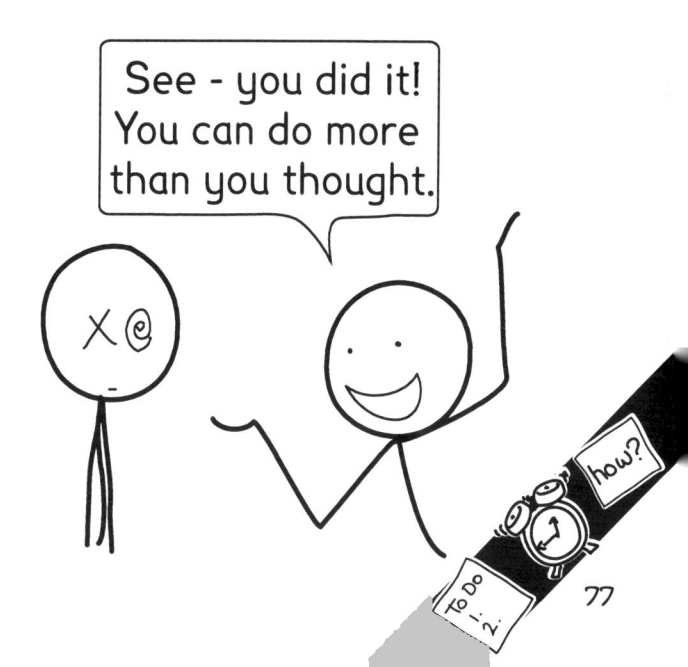

> See - you did it! You can do more than you thought.

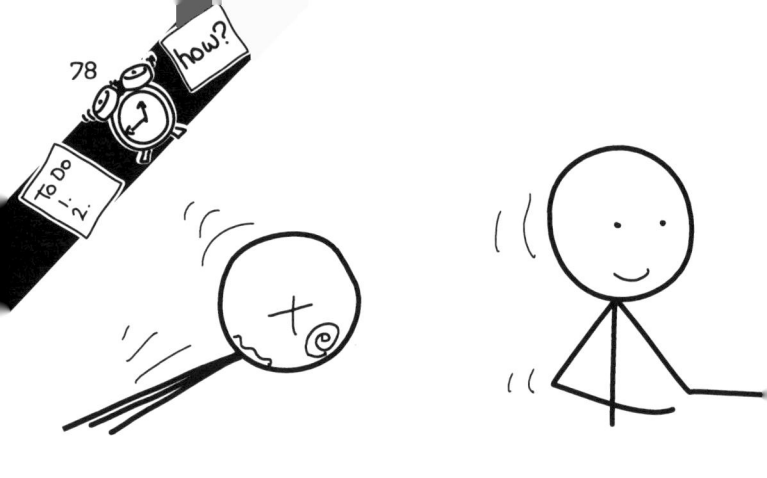

But if you don't let them see the effects, you may have accidentally communicated that they were right - you could do it when you thought you couldn't.

It's very hard for people who haven't personally experienced our condition to understand our limitations and challenges.

Make sure you let people who you spend a lot of time with, or are close to, see past the 'I'm okay' mask - into how you actually feel. If you hide your symptoms from them, they will never understand.

Answering "how are you?" with "fine" is OK sometimes, but it stops that person from learning how your condition affects you.

Finding a way to communicate about symptoms levels is important.

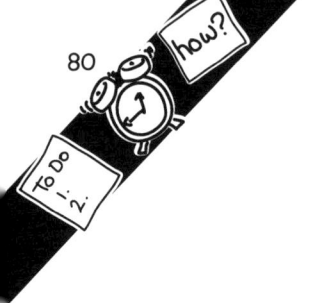

It can be hard to pace when people around you keep getting things so wrong....

They interfere with offers of help when you are fine...

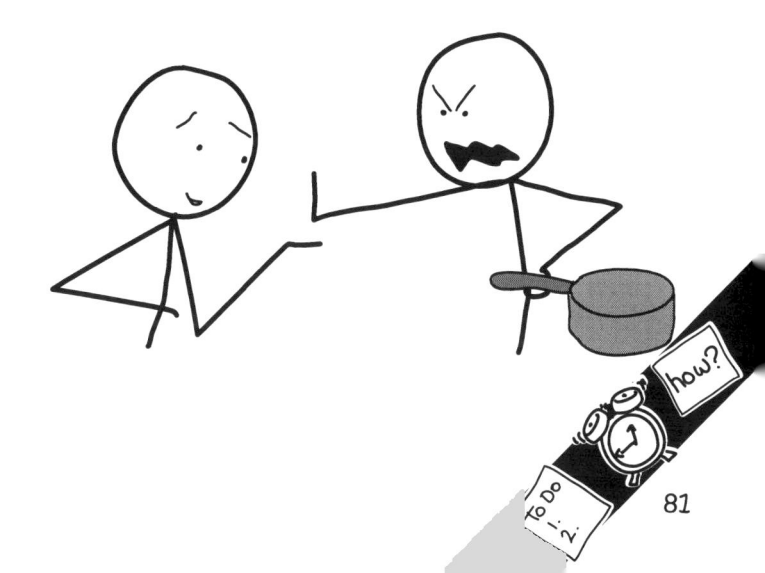

...and ignore you when you are desperate for help.

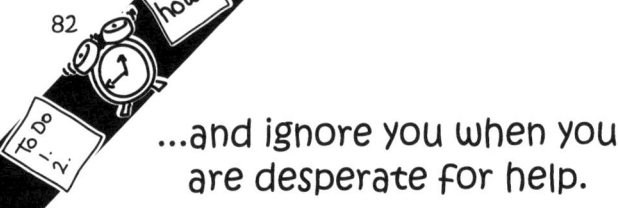

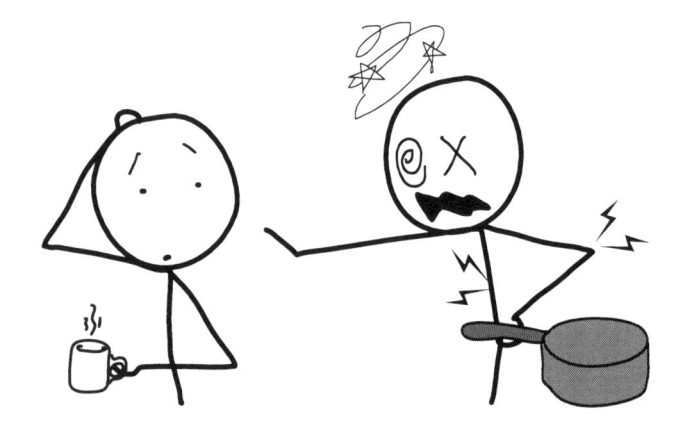

Fatigue and pain aren't visible in real life. People can't always see when help is needed, and often get it wrong. As a result everyone gets cross and frustrated.

Find a way to communicate about symptom levels which works for you.

Explain the issue when you aren't in the middle of a misunderstanding, have an agreed way of communicating how you are - a coloured wristband, a code word, a 'bad day' hoodie, a sign or badge - or whatever works for you.

Some people over-react when they hear "can't" in the context of hidden symptoms like pain and fatigue.

This may be why:

In medical-speak:
Can't = physical impossibility.

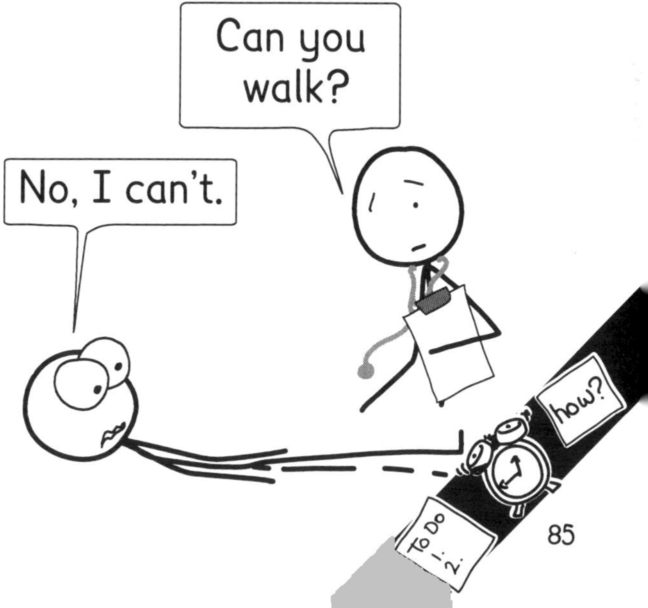

86

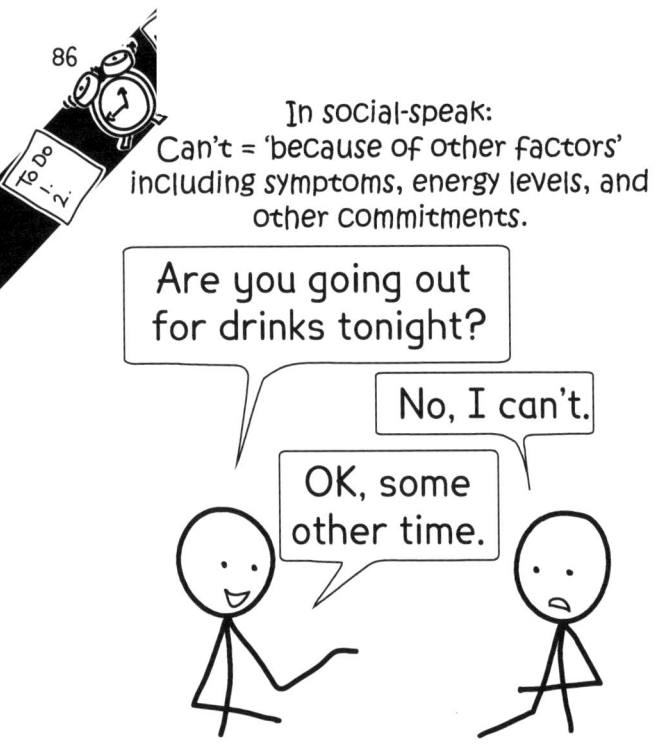

In social-speak:
Can't = 'because of other factors' including symptoms, energy levels, and other commitments.

Are you going out for drinks tonight?

No, I can't.

OK, some other time.

People with medical conditions often speak in 'social' - but are heard in medical, creating frustration and misunderstandings...

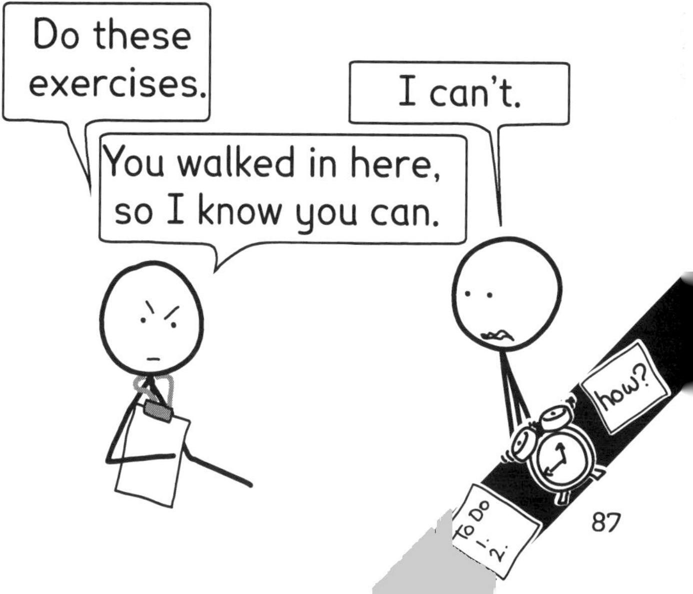

These might help communicate "can't".

1. People get scared we have given up - including a 'can' helps them understand that you haven't.
"I can't do it like that, I can do it like this".
Or "I'd love to, let's see if we can find a way for it to work."
Or "I can't. Can we do this instead?"

2. Give more info and a context that makes it clearer. For example "Last time I tried that, this happened".

3. You don't need to explain in detail. Focus on communicating the key point not all the background.

4. Be prepared for it to take time for people to accept can't. Sticking to your "No" and allowing others to see your symptoms and your coping mechanisms will help them be more accepting in the future.

5. Remember that through the internet you may be able to 'join in' remotely. A video-linked "Hi!" and short chat at an event you couldn't otherwise go to may be worth considering.

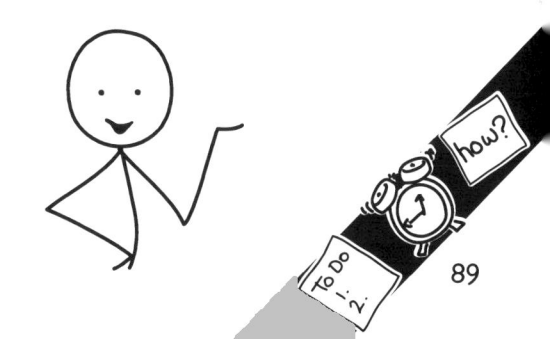

Timing

Most of us have times we pace well, and times we don't.

Pacing is easier to prioritise when symptoms are severe and it's the only way to get things done. When things are going well and we can cope with more, it can stop being top priority and symptoms can slowly start to get worse. Pacing also often goes a bit wrong when our condition or lifestyle* changes.

This is normal and we've all been there! Revisit the pacing basics, starting at getting to know your body, and the skills you learnt before will soon help you get back on track.

*e.g. New job, new family member, new house, new school.

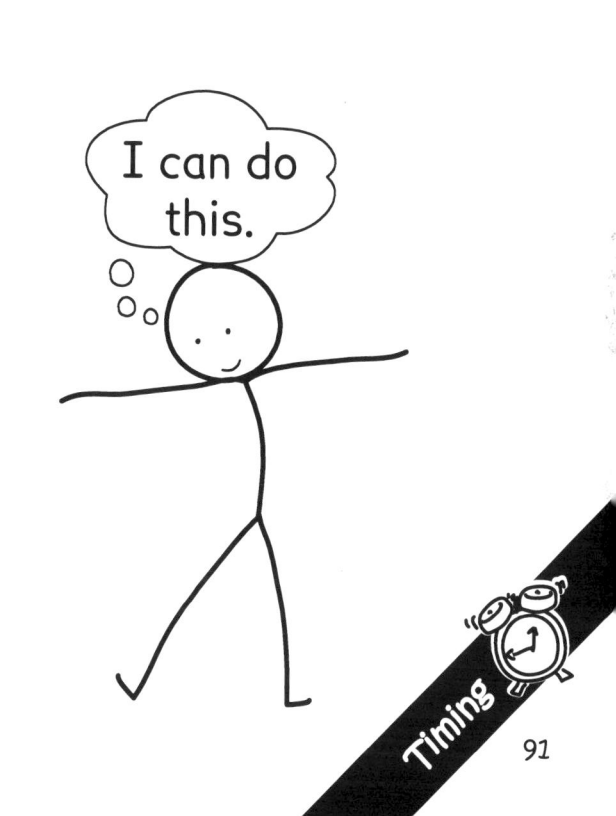

Pacing can be hard work.

It takes planning, saying no, changing habits, finding new ways of doing things, and lots of communicating.

But being able to live life in a way that works for us makes it all worthwhile.

93

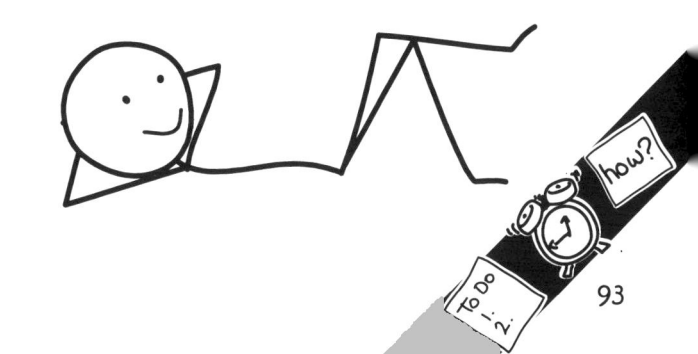

About the Author and Illustrator: Hannah Ensor

Hannah Ensor has a BSc (Hons) Environmental Health and worked in the field for 5 years before being medically retired at age 28 due to a hypermobility spectrum disorder (see hypermobility.org) and postural orthostatic tachycardia syndrome (see PoTSuk.org).

Meeting misunderstandings and metaphorical brick walls when communicating about her conditions, she looked for ways to open vital lines of communication - whether with friends and family, colleagues, or medical professionals. During a hospital stay where her ability to speak was very limited, she discovered that stickmen combined with straight forward, simple written explanations got the message across well.

This quickly developed into Stickman Communications®, a company using stickman cartoons to break down the barriers and communicate positively yet realistically about a wide range of disabilities, conditions, needs and symptoms. Her products, blogs, and talks are used worldwide by people with disabilities and medical professionals.

Alongside this she is an entertaining and insightful speaker, is featured in the 2016 and 2017 'Power 100' lists of Britain's most influential people with a disability or impairment, is a Trustee of The Hypermobility Syndromes Association, has worked various other charities including MIND, Whizz-Kidz and PoTS UK, and is a contemporary dancer.

Other useful resources

StickmanCommunications.co.uk has a range of other pacing tools including pacing sticky notes, scheduling fridge magnets, posters and more.

PainToolkit.org has some great pain management resources, including ones on pacing. All created by Pete Moore, who lives with persistent pain.